THE BASIC CONCEPT OF MEDICARE:

Guide to know the basic concept and benefits of medicare

Thomas Haigler

1

Table of contents

Chapter 1:Medicare

Medicare is a U.S. government health insurance program that subsidizes healthcare services. The plan covers persons age 65 or older, younger people who fulfill particular qualifying conditions, and those with certain disorders.

Medicare is separated into multiple plans that cover a range of healthcare situations—some of which come at a cost to the covered individual. While this enables the program to give customers greater options in terms of pricing and coverage, it also creates a complication for those looking to join up.

is the federal government program that offers health care coverage (health insurance) if you are 65+, under 65, and receiving Social Security Disability Insurance (SSDI) for a set length of time, or under 65 and having End-Stage Renal Disease (ESRD) (ESRD). The Centers for Medicare & Medicaid Services (CMS) is the government organization that manages Medicare. The program is supported in part by Social Security and Medicare taxes you pay on your income, in part by premiums that those with Medicare pay, and in part by the government budget.

Once you have become Medicare-eligible and enrolled, you can choose to get your Medicare benefits from Original Medicare, the traditional fee-for-service program offered directly through the federal government, or from a Medicare Advantage Plan, a type of private insurance offered by companies that contract with Medicare (the federal government) (the federal government).

It is vital to understand your Medicare coverage options and to select your plan wisely. How you choose to acquire your benefits and whom you get them from might affect your out-of-pocket expenditures and where you can get your treatment. For instance, with Original Medicare, you are insured to travel to practically all physicians and hospitals in the nation. Medicare Advantage Plans, on the other hand, frequently contain network limits, meaning that you will be more restricted in your access to physicians and hospitals. However, Medicare Advantage Plans may also offer extra services that Original Medicare does not cover, such as basic vision or dental care

Chapter 2:History

Discussion about a national health insurance system for Americans extends back to the days of President Teddy Roosevelt, whose platform included health insurance when he campaigned for president in 1912. But the notion of a national health plan didn't acquire pace until it was promoted by U.S. President Harry S Truman.

On November 19, 1945, seven months into his administration, Truman issued a letter to Congress, proposing the development of a national health insurance fund, available to all Americans. The plan Truman envisioned would give health coverage to people, paying for such common charges as doctor appointments, hospital visits, laboratory tests, dental care, and nursing services.
Although Truman pushed to get a measure approved during his administration, he was unsuccessful and it was another 20 years

before any sort of national health insurance — Medicare for Americans 65 and older, rather than previous ideas to cover eligible Americans of all ages – would become a reality.

President John F. Kennedy launched his own failed campaign for a national health care program for seniors after a nationwide survey indicated that 56 percent of Americans over the age of 65 were not covered by health insurance.

But it wasn't until after 1966 – after legislation was signed by President Lyndon B Johnson in 1965 – that Americans began obtaining Medicare health coverage when Medicare's hospital and medical insurance benefits initially took effect. Harry Truman and his wife, Bess, were the first two Medicare enrollees.

By August 2021, there were roughly 63.8 million individuals obtaining health coverage via Medicare. Medicare expenditure reached $926 billion in 2020 and accounted for around 21 percent of total national health spending in 2019.

Medicare expenditure forecasts change with time, but as of 2021, the Medicare Part A trust fund was predicted to be drained by 2026. (Medicare will continue to exist, but claims will have to be financed by payroll taxes, which won't be adequate to completely cover all Part A claims.)

But Medicare per capita expenditure has been expanding at a considerably slower rate in recent years, averaging 1.5 percent between 2010 and 2017, as compared to 7.3 percent between 2000 and 2007. Per capita expenditure is predicted to expand at a greater pace during the future decade, although not as rapidly as it did in the first decade of the 21st century.

A short look at Medicare milestones\sThe '60s

On July 30, 1965, President Lyndon B. Johnson made Medicare law by signing H.R. 6675 in Independence, Missouri. Former President Truman was awarded the very first Medicare card on the occasion. In 1965, the budget for Medicare was roughly $10 billion.
In 1966, Medicare's coverage took effect, when Americans age 65 and over were enrolled in Part A and millions of additional seniors joined up for Part B. Nineteen million persons joined up for Medicare within its first year.
The '70s

In 1972, President Richard M. Nixon put into law the first significant adjustment to Medicare. The Act increased coverage to include adults under the age of 65 with

long-term impairments and those with end-stage renal disease (ERSD) (ERSD). People with disabilities have to wait for Medicare coverage, while Americans with ESRD may obtain coverage as early as three months after they begin regular hospital dialysis treatments – or immediately if they go through a home-dialysis training program and begin conducting in-home dialysis. This has acted as a lifeline for Americans with renal failure - a severe and incredibly costly condition.
The '80s

When Congress approved the Omnibus Reconciliation Act of 1980, it increased home health care. The measure also placed Medigap – or Medicare supplement insurance – under government regulation.
In 1982, hospice services for the terminally sick were added to a growing list of Medicare benefits.
In 1988, Congress approved the Medicare Catastrophic Coverage Act, putting a real

limit to Medicare's total out-of-pocket payments for Part A and Part B, coupled with a restricted prescription drug benefit. Most of the Catastrophic Care statute was overturned less than a year later amid resistance from senior groups over the program's increased rates. (To this day, there remains to be no restriction on out-of-pocket expenditures for Medicare A and B.)

The new legislation also compelled states to "buy in" to the Medicare system by utilizing Medicaid monies to pay Medicare premiums and cost-sharing for disadvantaged Medicare enrollees. These people are known as Qualified Medicare Beneficiaries (QMB) (QMB). In 2016, there were 7.5 million Medicare beneficiaries who were QMBs, and Medicaid funds were being utilized to pay their Medicare premiums and cost-sharing. To be deemed a QMB, you have to be eligible for Medicare and have income that doesn't exceed 100 percent of the federal poverty line.

The '90s

The new law mandated state Medicaid programs to reimburse premiums of the new Specified Low-Income Medicare Beneficiary (SLMB) eligibility category — individuals eligible for Medicare with incomes between 100 and 120 percent of the federal poverty line.

Congress also approved the Qualified Individual (QI) programs and the surviving program (of two initially established) mandates Medicaid to pay premiums (via a federal grant) for Part B participants with earnings between 120 and 135 percent of poverty. The yearly budget for QI is limited and once gone, recipients are not eligible to receive the benefit — but governments may offer it at their own cost. Unlike QMB and SLMB, the QI program must be reauthorized by Congress every few years, and states normally do not take part in supporting it.

Other legislation allowed persons qualifying for Medicare coverage greater alternatives on the private market under Medicare Part C - Medicare Advantage (MA) (MA). Originally called Medicare HMOs or "Medicare+Choice" (among other titles), the new private choices finally provided add-on benefits such as prescription medication coverage for new subscribers. The Affordable Care Act mandates increased accountability from these plans, including connecting the insurers' payments to the star rating system — a gauge of many different ways the plans are obliged to offer excellent care.

The '00s

Americans younger than age 65 with amyotrophic lateral sclerosis (ALS) can enroll in Medicare without a waiting period if accepted for Social Security Disability Insurance (SSDI) income. (Most SSDI claimants have a 24-month waiting period for Medicare from when their disability cash payments start.)

President George W. Bush signed into law the Medicare Prescription Medication Improvement and Modernization Act of 2003, establishing an optional prescription drug coverage known as Part D, which is offered solely by private insurers. Until this moment, around 25 percent of Americans getting Medicare coverage did not have a prescription drug plan. Medicare Part D plans became available in 2006; Part D may be bought as a stand-alone plan, but it can also be linked with Medicare Advantage plans (90 percent of Medicare Advantage plans include Part D coverage as of 2019). (90 percent of Medicare Advantage plans include Part D coverage as of 2019). As of early 2019, more than 45 million Medicare beneficiaries —about three-quarters of the Medicare population — had Medicare Part D coverage (Medicare beneficiaries can also obtain prescription coverage from an employer or retiree program, or Medicaid if

they're eligible for both Medicare and Medicaid).
2010

The Patient Protection and Affordable Care Act of 2010 contains a large range of reform proposals aimed to reduce Medicare expenditures while boosting revenue, enhancing and simplifying its delivery systems, and even expanding services to the program.

Chapter 3: The four General parts

There are four main Parts of Medicare: A, B, C, and D. Then you have the 10 types of Medicare supplement plans: A, B, C, D, F, G, K, L, M, and N.

As complex as it can appear, it's crucial to take the time to educate yourself. Medicare's parts and supplement plans cover various things. They have various pricing; participating doctor and hospital networks; availability; and other criteria. You'll most likely be enrolled in many segments and/or plans at the same time. Getting acquainted with them enables you to select the finest health insurance for your requirements.

Part A: Hospital Services

Medicare Parts A and B are handled by a government body called the Centers for

Medicare and Medicaid Services. Together, these two elements are known as Original Medicare. With Original Medicare, you may visit any doctor or hospital anywhere in the nation — as long as they participate in the program and are accepting new Medicare patients. If you visit a non-participating doctor, your out-of-pocket expenditures rise.

Most individuals join up for Original Medicare during their first enrollment period. This is the 7-month period that begins 3 months before the month of your 65th birthday and concludes 3 months after.

OK, how about Part A specifically?

This is Medicare's program for sickness or injury severe enough to warrant treatment in a hospital or other health care institution. Generally, Part A covers:

- A hospital stay that a doctor thinks is required

- A stay in a skilled nursing facility or nursing home when such care is short-term, authorized by a doctor, and follows a hospital stay

- Home health care for treatments your doctor recommends, such as physical, occupational, and speech therapy

- Hospice treatment when physicians declare that you're anticipated to die within 6 months.

Most individuals can acquire Part A without paying a premium. If you or your spouse paid Medicare taxes for at least 10 years, you qualify for no-premium coverage. You can qualify if you obtain retirement payments from Social Security or the Railroad Retirement Board.

Part A does not pay your long-term care expenditures unless they are medically required

Part A is designed for inpatient treatment, don't make the mistake of believing that it will pay for assisted-living care or long-term care that wasn't recommended by your doctor.

Part B: Medical Services

Part B is Medicare's coverage for doctor visits, testing, and other outpatient services. It covers medically essential services and certain preventative ones, including checkups. It also may pay for:

- Participation in a clinical research study

- Ambulance travels (including some nonemergency journeys) (including some nonemergency trips)

- Durable" medical equipment like walkers or oxygen tanks

- Mental health care

- Certain prescription medications that are frequently provided by a doctor or at a hospital

With Part B, you pay:

A premium that might grow with your income, a deductible normally 20 percent of the price for each medical care (called coinsurance)
This highlights a key point: Original Medicare may be operated by the government, but that doesn't imply it's free to you.

"Medicare is typically greater coverage than you received from commercial insurance before age 65, but it is not free these days.

Even those of moderate resources face costs," adds Lina Walker, Ph.D., vice president of health security at the AARP's Public Policy Institute.

Also, bear in mind that sections A and B don't cover most dental care, eye examinations, hearing aids or tests to fit them, cosmetic surgery, acupuncture, or basic foot care. Parts A and B also don't cover most prescription medications. You need to enroll in a Part D or Medicare Advantage plan for that.

Part C: Medicare Advantage

If you want additional services like those — and are ready to pay more to receive them — Part C, or a Medicare Advantage plan, maybe for you.

These plans are just another method to acquire your Medicare benefits. They're offered by commercial insurance firms that are authorized by Medicare.

The plans must at least provide you with the same advantages as Part A and Part B. The private insurers then provide more services. In addition to visual, dental, and hearing care, they can include items like:

- A wellness program

- Adult day-care services

- Transportation to doctor

Most also provide the prescription medication coverage you'd normally obtain via Medicare Part D (more about that later) (more on that later).

With Part C, the government pays the insurance firm a predetermined sum every month for your treatment. But the firm determines your out-of-pocket payments.

You also deal with deductibles and coinsurance, just like you did with your employer's insurance.

Some Medicare Advantage plans also charge monthly premiums. If you enroll in one of them, you may pay it on top of your Part B premium. Some plans, nevertheless, cover all or part of your Part B premiums. You could hear this labeled the "give-back benefit."

Part D: Prescription Drugs

Maybe you don't want to join up for a Medicare Advantage plan, or the plans in your region don't provide the sort of medication coverage you need. You've got one more choice to explore: a private insurance company's Part D plan.

All Part D plans must include a spectrum of prescription pharmaceuticals that individuals with Medicare commonly use, including more specialist treatments like cancer therapies and insulin. Each Part D plan provides a list of its covered pharmaceuticals, termed a formulary. In each formulary, medications are grouped into multiple tiers with variable pricing.

Bear these considerations in mind with Part D plans:

- You must have Part A and Part B coverage to enroll in one.

- Drug coverage is optional. But if you don't sign up for Part D when you initially enroll in Medicare, you may face fines for enrolling later on.

- If you have medication coverage via your Medicare Advantage plan, you don't need a separate Part D plan.

Medicare Supplement Plans (Medigap)

Medigap, or Medicare supplement, plans are supplemental insurance to pay for all or part of the deductibles, coinsurance, and copayments you have with Original Medicare. You acquire them from private insurance firms.

Medigap, or Medicare supplement, plans are supplemental insurance to pay for all or part of the deductibles, coinsurance, and copayments you have with Original Medicare. You acquire them from private insurance firms.

There are 10 Medigap plans, which differ in what and how much they cover. Each is recognized by a letter: A, B, C, D, F, G, K, L, M, and N. They're standardized, which means a Plan A supplied by one firm has the same advantages as a Plan A sold by another one. Your premiums may vary, however. To see out what benefits are given under each plan, go to the Medicare website.

Each insurance company determines which Medigap policies it wants to market, while certain states' laws mandate them to provide particular plans there.

A few things to know regarding Medigap plans:

You'll continue paying your Part B rates, along with your Medigap premiums.

Each policy protects only one individual. Your partner will need a separate one if you both want coverage.

Those sold to those who are newly eligible for Medicare don't pay Part B deductibles. New participants haven't been able to purchase C or F Medigap plans since Jan. 1, 2020.

The optimum time to purchase one is when you're initially eligible. You'll likely confront fewer options and greater pricing if you attempt to acquire one later on.

Chapter 4: Eligibility

In general, people in the age range of 65 are eligible for Medicare if:

You are a U.S. citizen or a permanent legal resident who has resided in the United States for at least five years and

You are receiving Social Security or railroad retirement benefits or have worked long enough to be eligible for such benefits but are not yet collecting them.

You or your spouse is a government employee or retiree who has not paid into Social Security but has paid Medicare payroll taxes while working

Also, you may be eligible if you fall within the age range of 65 but only qualified if:

You have been eligible for Social Security disability payments for at least 24 months (that need not be consecutive); or

You get a disability pension from the Railroad Retirement Board and fulfill certain requirements; or

You have Lou Gehrig's illness, generally known as amyotrophic lateral sclerosis (ALS), which qualifies you instantly; or

You have persistent renal failure needing frequent dialysis or a kidney transplant — and you or your spouse has paid Social Security taxes for a set time, depending on your age.

Again, there are alternative options to receive Medicare coverage by buying into them through:

Paying premiums for Part A, the hospital insurance. How much you would have to pay for Part A depends on how long you've worked. The longer you labor, the more work credits you will earn. Work credits are earned depending on your income; the amount of money it takes to get a credit increases each year.

Paying the same monthly payments for Part B, which covers doctor visits and other outpatient services, that other participants pay.

Paying the same monthly payment for Part D prescription medication coverage as those enrolled in the drug plan you pick.

Chapter 5: Benefits

If you are nearing age 65, you may be beginning to think about the government benefits you will soon qualify for. For example, your healthcare choice to choose between Original Medicare or a Medicare Advantage plan.

Saves You Money

First and foremost, Medicare Advantage Plans save Medicare participants money –and not just a little bit of money, but a lot of money.

Original Medicare only covers 80 percent of the cost of medical treatment — the Medicare recipient is liable for the remaining 20 percent. A Medicare Advantage Plan is different. The Medicare

Beneficiary is only liable for a minimal copay, often less than 20 percent of a medical visit or treatment.

More crucially, Medicare Advantage Plans have a maximum out-of-pocket price, meaning that once you hit the limit, the Plan pays 100 percent of all medical expenses. That alone may save thousands of dollars every year - especially if there is a hospitalization involved.

Dental, Vision, and Hearing Coverage

What makes Medicare Advantage plans unique is the extra benefits that Original Medicare doesn't cover.
These benefits include dental treatment, eye coverage, hearing tests, and hearing aid coverage. None of these crucial health care benefits are covered in Original Medicare. Also, most Medicare Advantage Plans to provide prescription drug coverage at no

additional expense, but persons with Original Medicare need to sign-up and pay extra for Part D prescription drug coverage.

Medicare Advantage Plans provide greater benefits than Original Medicare and can help members save on their health care expenditures.

Focus on Accessibility, Wellness, and Preventative Health

Accessible healthcare coverage is crucial to remain on top of your health. To join a Medicare Advantage Plan you must have Part A and Part B coverage and reside in the plan's service region. It is vital to note that Original Medicare is only valid in the United States. Fortunately, many Medicare Advantage Plans include international emergency coverage.

Another key healthcare issue to bear in mind is Medicare Advantage Plans concentrate on your total well-being. They provide preventive and wellness-related advantages at no cost to you. This offers key perks like free over-the-counter medications and free gym memberships. You won't find those sorts of advantages with Original Medicare.

Medicare Supplement Plans (Medigap) (Medigap)

Some individuals mistake a Medicare Supplement Plan, often known as a Medigap Plan, with Medicare Advantage Plans. They are different and the largest distinction is Medicare Supplement plans come with ever-increasing rates since they are dependent on your age. This implies the cost of these plans grows every year. Plus, they don't give any extra benefit coverage like vision, dentistry, or hearing.

That's not the case with a Medicare Advantage Plan. In many circumstances, there is no monthly charge and you obtain all kinds of extra advantages. These benefit-rich, zero-dollar premium Medicare Advantage plans are persuading patients to say goodbye to expensive Medicare supplement plans and welcome to Medicare Advantage Plans.

Don't worry, if you join a Medicare Advantage Plan for the first time and you aren't content with the plan, you'll have unique rights under federal law to purchase Medigap insurance and a Medicare prescription plan if you return to Original Medicare within 12 months of joining the Medicare Advantage Plan.

The Flexibility to Change Your Mind

A widespread myth concerning Medicare Advantage Plans is that when you join, you are still on Medicare and are not giving up your Medicare coverage. Medicare Advantage Plans are designated "Medicare Part C." This means they combine your Medicare Part A (hospital coverage), Part B (doctor's coverage), and Part D (prescription drug coverage) into one easy plan that costs less and gives more.

www.ingramcontent.com/pod-product-compliance
Lightning Source LLC
Chambersburg PA
CBHW070231260726
48658CB00006BA/2283